The Green Way to Diet

Healthy and Simple Vegetarian Recipes to Lower Your Carbs Intake and Boost Your Metabolism

America Best Recipes

Table of Contents

Breakfast 6

  Green Colada 6

  Berry Beet Velvet Smoothie 7

  Strawberry, Banana and Coconut Shake 9

  Ginger and Greens Smoothie 10

  Chocolate Cherry Smoothie 11

  Crust Less Sweet Potato...12

  Spinach Muffins 14

  Nutmeg Buckwheat 16

  Porridge 18

  Honey-nutmeg Cereal Bowls 20

Lunch 22

  Keto Creamy Avocado Pasta with Shirataki.................22

  Spinach Artichoke Egg Casserole Recipe 24

  Zucchini Noodles Salad with Parmesan & Walnuts 26

  Easy Four Cheese Pesto Zoodles................................28

  Fathead Keto Gnocchi 31

  Low Carb Zucchini Lasagna Skillet 34

  Low Carb Spinach & Artichoke Dip Cauliflower Casserole 38

  Zucchini Noodles with Creamy Roasted Tomato Basil Sauce 40

  Keto Egg Fast Fettuccini Alfredo 42

  Low Carb Falafel with Tahini Sauce 45

Soups and Salads 48

  Crispy Tofu and Bok Choy Salad 48

  Low-Carb Snap Pea Salad...51

Black Bean Salad with Apricots.................................... 54

Red Potato Salad 56

Awesome Pasta Salad 58

Lemon-Mint Millet Salad 60

Beet and Carrot Barley Salad 62

Quinoa, Asparagus, and Cucumber Salad 64

Wild Rice Salad with Tofu 66

Buckwheat Salad with Mint, Walnuts, and Cranberries.... 68

Dinner 70

Peanut Chutney Mushrooms with Tamarind 70

Tofu with 20 Cloves of Garlic....................................... 74

Mushrooms and Olive Curry 76

Baked Kohlrabi Yucca Root and Mustard Greens............ 79

Baked Brussel Sprouts & Red Onion Glazed with Balsamic
Vinegar 80

Roasted Microgreens and Potatoes............................... 83

Roasted Spinach & Broccoli with Jalapeno 85

Spicy Baked Swiss Chard and Cauliflower...................... 87

Thai Carrots and Collard Greens 89

Baked White Yam and Spinach 91

Sweets.. 93

Carrot Oatmeal Muffins 93

Banana Blueberry Muffins.. 95

Lemon Zucchini Muffins... 97

Banana Chocolate Chip Muffins.................................... 99

Brownie Muffins 101

Milkshake ice pops 103

Whisky & pink peppercorn marmalade kit Easy 104

Simnel muffins 105

Prunes Cake.. 107

Butternut squash. -Almond Cookies 109

Breakfast

Green Colada

Preparation time: 5 minutes Cooking time: 0 minute

Servings: 1

Ingredients:

1/2 cup frozen pineapple chunks

1/2 banana

1/2 teaspoon spirulina powder

1/4 teaspoon vanilla extract, unsweetened

1 cup of coconut milk

Directions:

Place all the ingredients in the order in a food processor or blender and then pulse for 2 to 3 minutes at high speed until smooth. Pour the smoothie into a glass and then serve.

Berry Beet Velvet Smoothie

Preparation time: 5 minutes Cooking time: 0 minute

Servings: 1

Ingredients:

1/2 of frozen banana

1 cup mixed red berries

1 Medjool date, pitted

1 small beet, peeled, chopped

1 tablespoon cacao powder

1 teaspoon chia seeds

1/4 teaspoon vanilla extract, unsweetened

1/2 teaspoon lemon juice

2 teaspoons coconut butter

1 cup coconut milk, unsweetened

Directions:

Place all the ingredients in the order in a food processor or blender and then pulse for 2 to 3 minutes at high speed until smooth. Pour the smoothie into a glass and then serve.

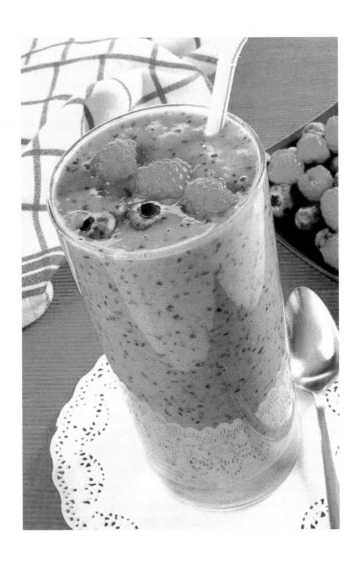

Strawberry, Banana and Coconut Shake

Preparation time: 5 minutes Cooking time: 0 minute

Servings: 1

Ingredients:

1 tablespoon coconut flakes

1 1/2 cups frozen banana slices

8 strawberries, sliced

1/2 cup coconut milk, unsweetened

1/4 cup strawberries for topping

Directions:

Place all the ingredients in the order in a food processor or blender, except for topping and then pulse for 2 to 3 minutes at high speed until smooth. Pour the smoothie into a glass and then serve.

Ginger and Greens Smoothie

Preparation time: 5 minutes Cooking time: 0 minute

Servings: 1

Ingredients:

1 frozen banana

2 cups baby spinach

2-inch piece of ginger, peeled, chopped

¼ teaspoon cinnamon

¼ teaspoon vanilla extract, unsweetened

1/8 teaspoon salt

1 scoop vanilla protein powder

1/8 teaspoon cayenne pepper

2 tablespoons lemon juice 1 cup of orange juice

Directions:

Place all the ingredients in the order in a food processor or blender and then pulse for 2 to 3 minutes at high speed until smooth. Pour the smoothie into a glass and then serve.

Chocolate Cherry Smoothie

Preparation time: 5 minutes Cooking time: 0 minute

Servings: 1

Ingredients:

1 1/2 cups frozen cherries, pitted

1 cup spinach

1/2 small frozen banana

2 tablespoon cacao powder, unsweetened

1 tablespoon chia seeds

1 scoop of vanilla protein powder

1 teaspoon spirulina

1 1/2 cups almond milk, unsweetened

Directions:

Place all the ingredients in the order in a food processor or blender and then pulse for 2 to 3 minutes at high speed until smooth. Pour the smoothie into a glass and then serve.

Crust Less Sweet Potato

Prep time: 20 min Cooking Time: 10 min Serve: 2

Ingredients

2 large eggs

2/8 cup almond milk

½ tsp parsley

1/8 tsp salt

1/16 tsp black pepper

1 tomato

1/8 cup potato

2 tbsp goat cheese

1 tbsp red onion

2 cups water

Cooking oil

Directions

In a bowl, whisk eggs, almond milk, parsley, salt, and pepper. Stir in tomato, sweet potato, goat cheese, and onion.

Add egg mixture to a glass dish greased with oil.

Add water to the Instant Pot. Place dish with egg mixture on steam rack.

Let pressure release naturally for 10 minutes.

Remove dish from pot and let sit 10 minutes. Slice and serve warm.

Nutrition Facts

Calories 190, Total Fat 13.7g, Saturated Fat 8.2g, Cholesterol 201mg , Sodium 283mg, Total Carbohydrate 6.1g, Dietary Fiber 1.4g , Total Sugars 3.3g, Protein 11.6g

Spinach Muffins

Prep time: 10 min Cooking Time: 10 min Serve: 2

Ingredients

½ teaspoon olive oil

1 cup spinach, finely chopped

¼ teaspoon salt

1/8 teaspoon ground black pepper

2 large eggs

2 tablespoons coconut cream

4 tablespoons shredded parmesan cheese optional

1 cup of water

Instructions

Use the ¼ teaspoon olive oil to grease the bottom and insides of two silicone muffin cups.

Set the Instant Pot to Sauté. Add the chopped spinach, salt and pepper. Sauté until the spinach is wilted, 2 to 3 minutes longer.

Meanwhile, in a medium bowl, gently beat the eggs, coconut cream, salt, and pepper.

Press Cancel. Divide the spinach mixture among the two muffin cups. Pour the egg mixture evenly over the spinach and stir lightly with a fork. If desired, top each with shredded cheese. Loosely cover the cups with foil or silicone lids.

Pour the water into the Instant Pot. Place the trivet inside. Place the two muffin cups on top.

Press the Pressure Cooker or Manual button and set the cook time to 5 minutes.

When the Instant Pot beeps, allow the pressure to release naturally for 10 minutes, then carefully switch the steam release valve to Venting.

Carefully remove the muffins from the Instant Pot.

Serve hot or warm.

Nutrition Facts

Calories 161, Total Fat 12.5g, Saturated Fat 6.6g, Cholesterol 193mg , Sodium 548mg, Total Carbohydrate 2.2g, Dietary Fiber 0.7g , Total Sugars 1g, Protein 10.9g

Nutmeg Buckwheat

Prep time: 10 min Cooking Time: 20 min Serve: 2

Ingredients

½ tablespoon butter

¼ cup buckwheat

2 cups water

1/8 teaspoon kosher salt

1 tablespoon maple syrup

½ teaspoon nutmeg

½ cup coconut cream

3/4 cup raisins

Instructions

Combine butter, water, buckwheat, salt, coconut cream, nutmeg, maple syrup in an Instant Pot. 2. Lock lid in place and turn the valve to Sealing.

Press the Pressure Cooker button and set the cook time for 5 minutes at High Pressure.

Open the Instant Pot to use natural pressure release.

Add raisins and nutmeg as topping.

Nutrition Facts

Calories 426, Total Fat 18.2g, Saturated Fat 14.7g, Cholesterol 8mg , Sodium 191mg, Total Carbohydrate 68.8g, Dietary Fiber 5.8g , Total Sugars 40.2g, Protein 5.9g

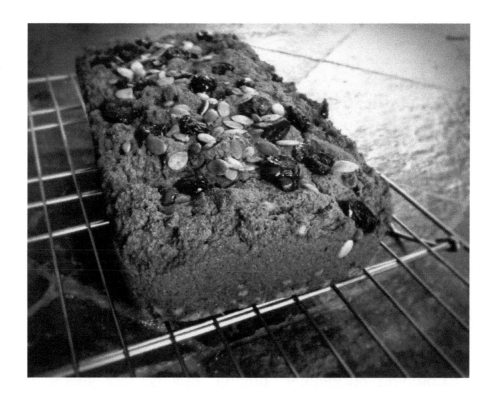

Porridge

Prep time: 10 min Cooking Time: 15 min Serve: 2

Ingredients

½ cup quinoa

1/8 cup uncooked buckwheat rinsed and drained

1/8 cup raisins

1 1/2 tablespoons ground flax seeds

1 tablespoon chia seeds

½ teaspoon butter

1/8 teaspoon salt

1/16 teaspoon ground nutmeg

1 1/2 cups coconut milk plus additional for serving

1 cup of water

Honey

Instructions

Combine buckwheat, quinoa, raisins, flax seeds, chia seeds, butter, salt and nutmeg in a non-stick bowl; mix well. Stir in coconut milk until blended.

Pour water into Instant Pot, then place bowl on rack in instant pot.

Press the Pressure Cooker button and set the cook time for 15 minutes at High Pressure.

When cooking is complete, use a natural pressure release.

Stir porridge until smooth. Serve with additional coconut milk, raisins, honey.

Nutrition Facts

Calories 573, Total Fat 34.8g, Saturated Fat 26.7g, Cholesterol 3mg, Sodium 181mg, Total Carbohydrate 59.9g, Dietary Fiber 9.2g , Total Sugars 18.1g, Protein 11.7g

Honey-nutmeg Cereal Bowls

Prep time:7 min Cooking Time: 10 min Serve: 2

Ingredients

1 cup quinoa

1 1/2 cups water

½ teaspoon ground nutmeg

1/8 cup honey

¼ teaspoon vanilla extract

1/8 teaspoon fine sea salt

Soy milk for serving

Chopped or sliced fresh fruit of choice

Instructions

Drain and rinse the quinoa, then combine it with the water, nutmeg, honey, vanilla extract, and salt in the Instant Pot and lock lid. Set the steam release valve to Sealing and select Manual/Pressure Cooker to cook at High Pressure for 10 minutes.

Let the pressure naturally release for 10 minutes. When the floating valve drops, carefully remove the lid and stir the cooked grains.

Serve the quinoa right away with soy milk and fresh fruit.

Nutrition Facts

Calories 390, Total Fat 5.6g, Saturated Fat 0.8g, Cholesterol 0mg , Sodium 134mg, Total Carbohydrate 73.3g, Dietary Fiber 6.2g , Total Sugars 18.2g, Protein 12.6g

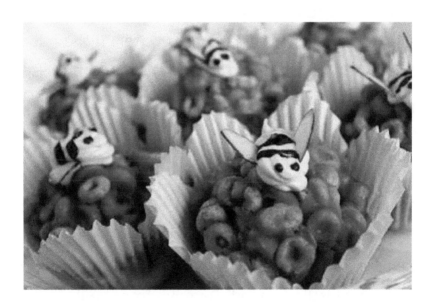

Lunch
Keto Creamy Avocado Pasta with Shirataki
Servings: 4

Ingredients

1 packet of shirataki noodles 1 avocado ripe

1/4 cup heavy cream 1 tsp dried basil

1 tsp black pepper 1 tsp salt

Instructions

Prepare the shirataki. Drain the shirataki noodles in a colander to remove the liquid they come packaged in. Rinse thoroughly under running water. If the noodles are rather long, cut into shorter pieces with scissors.

Boil some water and cook the shirataki for 1-2 mins to remove any lingering fragrance. Drain and rinse again.

Heat a clean dry frying pan and throw in the shirataki. The noodles contain large amounts of water, so this will help dry them out to remove some of their gelatinous texture. Cook for about a minute until they start to make a whistling sound. Remove from heat.

Prepare the sauce

In a bowl, mash your avocado and add the cream, basil, salt, and pepper. For a smoother texture, blend ingredients in a food processor.

Add to the frying pan with your shirataki noodles and stir through.

Serve hot with cheese and enjoy!

Nutrition Info

Calories: 453kcal Net carbs: 6g Carbs: 16g

Fibre: 10g Fat: 42g Protein: 4g Sugar: 3g

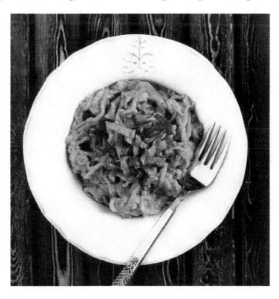

Spinach Artichoke Egg Casserole Recipe

Prep Time: 10 minutes Cook Time: 35 minutes Total Time: 45 minutes Servings: 12 servings

Ingredients

16 large eggs

1/4 cup milk

14 ounces artichoke hearts, 1 can drained

10 ounces frozen chopped spinach, 1 box thawed and drained well

1 cup shredded white cheddar 1/2 cup parmesan cheese

1/2 cup ricotta cheese 1/4 cup onion, shaved 1 clove garlic, minced 1 teaspoon salt

1/2 teaspoon dried thyme

1/2 teaspoon crushed red pepper

Instructions

Preheat the oven to 350 degrees F and spray a 9 X 13-inch baking dish with nonstick cooking spray. Crack the eggs into a large bowl and add the milk. Whisk the eggs well to combine. Break the artichoke hearts up into small pieces and separate the leaves. Squeeze the spinach with paper towels to remove all excess liquid. Then add both the artichokes and the spinach to the egg mixture. Add all remaining ingredients, withholding the ricotta cheese, and stir to combine. Pour the mixture into the prepared dish. Dollop the ricotta cheese evenly over the surface of the egg casserole. (I usually add about 12 dollops of ricotta, then break them in half with a spoon and separate them a little, so there are 24 "pockets" of ricotta throughout the mixture.) Place in the oven and bake for 30-35 minutes, until the center of the pan is fully cooked and doesn't jiggle when you shake the pan. Serve warm!

Nutrition Info

Calories: 230kcal Carbohydrates: 4g Protein: 16g Fat: 16g Saturated Fat: 6g Cholesterol: 300mg Sodium: 578mg Potassium: 222mg Fiber: 1g, Sugar: 1g

Zucchini Noodles Salad with Parmesan & Walnuts

A healthy alternative to pasta salad using low carb zucchini noodles. Loaded with Parmesan, walnuts, radicchio and parsley in a light lemon vinaigrette.

Servings: Four 1.5

Ingredients

For the salad:

4 cups spiralized zucchini noodles

1 cup fresh radicchio, shredded

1/4 cup fresh parsley, roughly chopped

1 oz parmesan cheese, shaved

1/4 cup walnuts, roughly chopped

For the vinaigrette:

1/3 cup avocado oil (or light olive oil)

1/4 cup fresh lemon juice

1 tsp minced fresh garlic

Instructions

1/2 tsp granulated sugar substitute (I used swerve)

Kosher salt and pepper to taste

Gently toss the salad ingredients together in a medium bowl. In a small bowl, whisk to together the vinaigrette ingredients. Pour the vinaigrette over the salad and toss gently to coat. Serve immediately.

Nutrition Info

265 calories 25g fat

5.5g net carbs 6g protein

Easy Four Cheese Pesto Zoodles

Perfect as a main meal or a side dish, this easy four cheese pesto zoodles recipe will win over even the pickiest of eaters with it's creamy texture and so. much.

Prep Time: 5 minutes Cook Time: 15 minutes Total Time: 20 minutes Servings: 4

Ingredients

8 ounces Mascarpone cheese

1/4 cup grated parmesan cheese

1/4 cup grated romano cheese

1/2 teaspoon kosher salt

1/4 teaspoon ground black pepper

1/8 teaspoon ground nutmeg

1/4 cup basil pesto (store-bought or homemade)

8 cups raw zucchini noodles (aka. spiral cut zucchini)

1 cup grated mozzarella cheese

Instructions

Preheat the oven to 400 degrees Fahrenheit.

Microwave the zucchini noodles uncovered, on high, for 3 minutes. Transfer to a colander lined with paper towels and gently squeeze out any moisture from the zoodles. Set aside.

In a large microwave safe bowl, combine the mascarpone cheese, parmesan cheese, Romano cheese, salt, pepper, and nutmeg. Microwave on high for 1 minute. Stir. Microwave on high for 30 more seconds.

Remove and whisk together until smooth.

Fold in the pesto and mozzarella cheese until fully incorporated.

Add the cooked zoodles and stir until well coated.

Transfer to a 2 quart casserole dish and bake in the oven for 10 minutes or until the cheese is bubbling at the edges. Remove and serve immediately.

Nutrition Info

Serving Size: 1 1/2 cups

Calories: 475 Fat: 43g

Carbohydrates: 8g Fiber: 3g

Protein: 13g

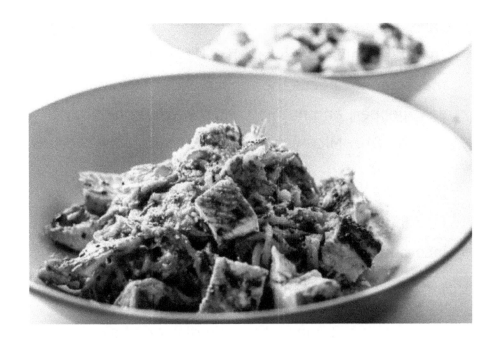

Fathead Keto Gnocchi

This Fathead Keto Gnocchi gives you the pillowy yet chewy texture you've been missing from pasta on a low carb diet! This keto gnocchi is the perfect low carb vehicle for all of your favorite pasta sauces and flavors!

Servings: 5 servings

Ingredients

For the keto gnocchi dough:

2 cups super fine blanched almond flour

2 cups shredded full fat mozzarella cheese 1/4 cup butter

1 large egg

1 large egg yolk

For the sauce:

1/4 cup salted butter 1 tsp lemon zest

1 tsp fresh thyme leaves

For the Fathead Keto Gnocchi:

Combine the mozzarella cheese and butter in a medium bowl and microwave for 2 minutes.

Stir, then microwave another minute.

Stir vigorously with a rubber spatula until thoroughly combined, and then cool for 2 minutes.

Stir in the egg, egg yolk and almond flour.

Continue to mix until a rough dough is formed, this could take several minutes.

Turn out the dough onto a smooth surface (or parchment paper) and knead until a semi-stretchy dough is formed. (if the dough is too wet, add a tablespoon or more of almond flour until workable)

Form the dough into a long roll about 1 inch in diameter and then cut pieces about 1/2" wide. You can then form them into almost any bite sized shape you want, but sticking with a simple disk as shown in the photos Servingsed the best results for me.

Freeze the gnocchi for 15 minutes to firm them up. before cooking, or freeze them until ready to eat.

Bring a pot of salted water to a gentle boil – too vigorous and the gnocchi will fall apart.

Add the gnocchi to the water in small batches and boil for 1 – 2 minutes or until floating.

Remove the gnocchi with a slotted spoon onto a paper towel lined plate, and cool for 5 minutes before adding to sauce.

For the sauce:

Melt the butter in a large saute pan. Add lemon zest and thyme and cook for about 2 minutes or until fragrant.

Add the boiled and cooled keto gnocchi to the pan and cook for about 2 minutes, stirring gently to coat with the sauce.

Season with salt and pepper as desired.

Nutrition Info

Serving Size: 1.5 cups Calories: 497

Fat: 44g Carbohydrates: 6g net Protein: 22g

Low Carb Zucchini Lasagna Skillet

This cheesy and saucy Low-Carb Zucchini Lasagna Skillet is a one-pan meal that has a delicious sauté mushroom filling, which brings this gluten-free lasagna to a new level of flavor. It's also very simple to assemble in a skillet.

Prep Time: 20 minutes Cook Time: 50 minutes

Total Time: 1 hour 10 minutes

Servings: 8 people

Ingredients

3 medium zucchini - sliced 16 oz mushroom - sliced

1   tbsp extra-virgin olive oil 15 oz part-skim ricotta

2   tbsp parsley - chopped

1 large egg

½ cup freshly grated Parmesan cheese

16 ounces part-skim mozzarella cheese - shredded

4 cups homemade tomato sauce - or sugar-free tomato sauce.

Instructions

Using a mandolin or sharp knife, slice the zucchini length-wise into long and thin slices (about 1/4-inch thick).

Then layer paper towels on your countertop. Spread the zucchini slices and sprinkle them with kosher salt.

Wait for 10-15 minutes to allow the excess liquid to be absorbed. Pat dry. (This step is very important to make before assembling your lasagna because it will help to draw out the moisture!)

Preheat oven to 375°.

In a skillet, heat olive oil over medium heat.

Add mushrooms and cook 5-7 minutes until they are soft and golden.

Add garlic and sauté for 30 seconds, being careful not to burn. Remove from the heat and set aside.

In a medium bowl, mix ricotta cheese, parmesan cheese, and an egg. Stir well.

Using the same skillet you sautéed the mushrooms, spread some tomato sauce on the bottom.

Layer 6 or 7 zucchini slices to cover.

Place some of the ricotta cheese mixture and top with the mozzarella cheese.

Add again another layer of tomato sauce and then add the mushrooms.

Repeat the layers until all your ingredients are all used up. Top with sauce and mozzarella.

Bake 40 minutes covered and 10 minutes uncovered. Let stand about 15 minutes before serving.

Garnish with parsley.

Nutrition Info

Calories: 294kcal Carbohydrates: 15g Protein: 23g

Fat: 16g Saturated Fat: 9g

Polyunsaturated Fat: 1g Monounsaturated Fat: 5g

Cholesterol: 71mg Sodium: 857mg Potassium: 556mg

Fiber: 3g

Sugar: 6g

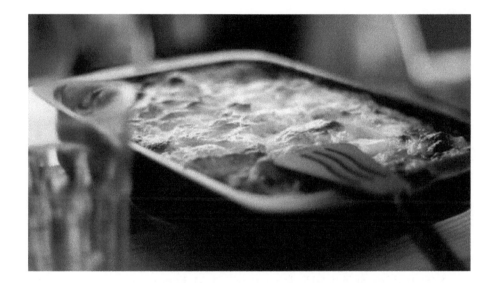

Low Carb Spinach & Artichoke Dip Cauliflower Casserole

A delicious low carb side dish recipe that can be turned into a main dish by adding some cooked chicken, or a breakfast or brunch recipe if you add some eggs!

Servings: 8 servings

Ingredients

4 cups raw cauliflower florets, roughly chopped 1/4 cup butter

1/2 cup Silk Cashew Milk, Unsweetened Original 8 oz full fat cream cheese

1/2 tsp kosher salt

1/8 tsp ground black pepper 1/4 tsp ground nutmeg

1/4 tsp garlic powder

1/4 tsp smoked paprika (use regular if you can't find smoked) 1 cup frozen, chopped spinach

3/4 cup canned or frozen artichoke hearts, drained and chopped 1 1/2 cup shredded whole milk mozzarella cheese

1/4 cup grated parmesan cheese

Instructions

Combine the cauliflower, butter, Silk Cashew Milk, cream cheese, salt, pepper, nutmeg, garlic powder, and paprika in a microwave safe dish. Microwave on high for ten minutes. Alternatively you could simmer it in a saucepan on the stove until the cauliflower is just fork tender. Add the spinach, artichoke hearts 1 cup of the shredded mozzarella, and the parmesan cheese to the cauliflower mixture and stir gently to combine thoroughly. Spoon the mixture into an ovenproof casserole dish and sprinkle the remaining 1/2 cup of mozzarella over the top. Bake for 20 minutes at 400 degrees (F) or until golden and bubbling. Serve hot.

Nutrition Info

252 calories 21g fat

4.5g net carbs 10g protein

Zucchini Noodles with Creamy Roasted Tomato Basil Sauce

These zucchini noodles with creamy roasted tomato basil sauce are the perfect way to enjoy fresh summer produce.

Prep Time: 5 minutes Cook Time: 30 minutes Total Time: 35 minutes Servings: 4 servings

Ingredients

2 pints grape tomatoes

2 tablespoons extra virgin olive oil salt and pepper

2 ounces cream cheese 1/4 cup fresh basil leaves

1/2 teaspoon red pepper flakes

2 large zucchini made into noodles with a julienne peeler or spiralizer

Instructions

Preheat oven to 400 degrees.

Toss tomatoes with olive oil, salt and pepper on a baking sheet. Roast in the oven for 20-30 minutes until the tomatoes start to brown and blister.

Remove the tomatoes from the oven and transfer to a food processor.

Add the cream cheese, basil, red pepper flakes, salt and pepper to taste and process until smooth.

Place zucchini noodles in a large bowl. Add the tomato sauce to the bowl and toss until all the noodles are coated.

Serve with freshly grated parmesan cheese.

Nutrition Info

Calories: 98 Total Fat: 8g

Carbohydrates: 5g Protein: 2g

Keto Egg Fast Fettuccini Alfredo

A low carb and gluten free Keto Egg Fast Fettuccini Alfredo recipe that is also keto, lchf, egg fast, and Atkins diet friendly!

Servings: 1 serving

Ingredients

For the pasta:

2 eggs

1 oz cream cheese pinch of salt

pinch of garlic powder 1/8 tsp black pepper

For the sauce:

1 oz Mascarpone cheese

1 Tbsp grated parmesan cheese 1 Tbsp butter

Instructions

For the pasta:

Blend the eggs, cream cheese, salt, garlic powder, and pepper in a magic bullet or blender. Pour into a butter-greased 8 x 8 pan. Bake at 325 for 8 minutes or until just set. Remove and let cool for about 5 minutes. Using a spatula, gently release the sheet of "pasta" from the pan. Roll it up and slice with a sharp knife into 1/8 inch thick slices. Gently unroll and set aside.

For the sauce:

Combine the mascarpone, parmesan cheese, and butter in a small bowl. Microwave on high for 30 seconds. Whisk. Microwave on high another 30 seconds. Whisk again until smooth (this may take a minute because the sauce will have separated – keep whisking and it will come back together!) Add the pasta to the hot sauce and toss gently. Serve immediately with more freshly ground black pepper if desired.

Alternative Sauce Recipe:

As an alternative to the mascarpone, you can make this sauce in the same method with 2 oz cream cheese, 2 Tbsp heavy whipping cream, 1 Tbsp parmesan, 1 Tbsp butter – it will taste amazing, but is not technically legal on the Egg Fast due to the heavy whipping cream. I doubt it will make a big difference in your results though, so if it's what you have on hand, go for it!

Nutrition Info

Calories: 491 Fat: 47g

Carbohydrates: 2g net Protein: 19g

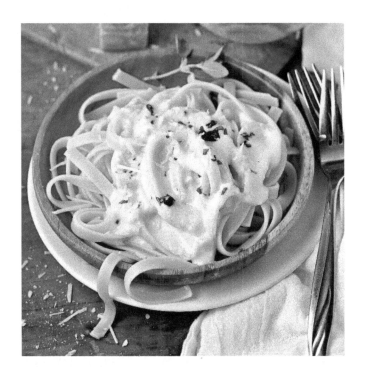

Low Carb Falafel with Tahini Sauce

Servings: (8) 3" patties

Ingredients

1   cup raw cauliflower, pureed 1/2 cup ground slivered almonds 1 Tbsp ground cumin

1/2 Tbsp ground coriander 1 tsp kosher salt

1/2 tsp cayenne pepper 1 clove garlic, minced

2   Tbsp fresh parsley, chopped 2 large eggs

3   Tbsp coconut flour

Tahini sauce:

2 Tbsp tahini paste 3 Tbsp water

1 Tbsp lemon juice

1 clove garlic, minced

1/2 tsp kosher salt, more to taste if desired

Instructions

For the cauliflower, you should end up with a cup of the puree. It takes about 1 medium head (florets only) to get that much. First chop it up with a knife, then add it to a food processor or magic bullet and pulse until it's blended but still has a grainy texture.

You can grind the almonds in a similar manner – just don't over grind them, you want the texture.

Combine the ground cauliflower and ground almonds in a medium bowl. Add the rest of the ingredients and stir until well blended.

Heat a half and half mix of olive and grapeseed (or any other light oil) oil until sizzling. While it's heating, form the mix into 8 three-inch patties that are about the thickness of a hockey puck.

Fry them four at a time until browned on one side and then flip and cook the other side. Resist the urge to flip too soon – you should see the edges turning brown before you attempt it – maybe 4 minutes or so per side. Remove to a plate lined with a paper towel to drain any excess oil.

Serve with tahini sauce and a tomato & parsley garnish if desired.

Tahini sauce: Blend all ingredients in a bowl. Thin with more water if you like a lighter consistency.

Nutrition Info

Serving Size: 2 patties Calories: 281

Fat: 24g Carbohydrates: 5g net Protein: 8g

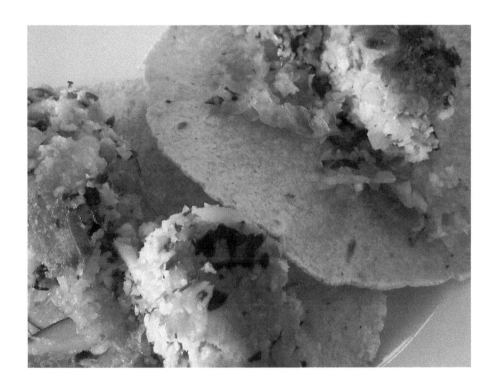

Soups and Salads

Crispy Tofu and Bok Choy Salad

Servings 3 servings

Ingredients

Oven Baked Tofu

15 ounces extra firm tofu

1 tablespoon soy sauce

1   tablespoon sesame oil

1 tablespoon water

2   teaspoons minced garlic

1 tablespoon rice wine vinegar

Juice ½ lemon

Bok Choy Salad

9 ounces bok choy

1 stalk green onion

2 tablespoons chopped cilantro

48

3 tablespoons coconut oil

2 tablespoons soy sauce 1 tablespoon sambal olek

1 tablespoon peanut butter

Juice ½ lime

7 drops liquid stevia

Instructions

Start by pressing the tofu. Lay the tofu in a kitchen towel and put something heavy over the top (like a cast iron skillet). It takes about 4-6 hours to dry out, and you may need to replace the kitchen towel half-way through.

Once the tofu is pressed, work on your marinade. Combine all of the ingredients for the marinade (soy sauce, sesame oil, water, garlic, vinegar, and lemon).

Chop the tofu into squares and place in a plastic bag along with the marinade. Let this marinate for at least 30 minutes, but preferably over night.

Pre-heat oven to 350°F. Place tofu on a baking sheet lined with parchment paper (or a silpat) and bake for 30-35 minutes.

As the tofu is cooked, get started on the bok choy salad. Chop cilantro and spring onion.

Mix all of the other ingredients together (except lime juice and bok choy) in a bowl. Then add cilantro and spring onion. Note: You can microwave coconut oil for 10-15 seconds to allow it it to melt.

Once the tofu is almost cooked, add lime juice into the salad dressing and mix together.

Chop the bok choy into small slices, like you would cabbage. Remove the tofu from the oven and assemble your salad with tofu, bok choy, and sauce. Enjoy!

Low-Carb Snap Pea Salad

This Low-Carb Snap Pea Salad makes a perfect side dish for Spring. It is suitable for low-carb, Atkins, LC/HF, gluten-free, and Banting diets.

Prep Time 5 minutes Cook Time 10 minutes Total Time 40 minutes Servings 4

Ingredients

8 ounces cauliflower riced

1/4 cup lemon juice

1/4 cup olive oil

1 clove garlic crushed

1/2 teaspoon coarse grain dijon mustard

1 teaspoon granulated stevia/erythritol blend

1/4 teaspoon pepper

1/2 teaspoon sea salt

1/2 cup sugar snap peas ends removed and each pod cut into three pieces

1/4 cup chives

1/2 cup sliced almonds 1/4 cup red onions minced

Instructions

Pour 1 to 2 inches of water in a pot fitted with a steamer. Bring water to a simmer.

Place riced cauliflower in the steamer basket, sprinkle lightly with sea salt, cover, and place over the simmering water in the bottom of the steamer. Steam until tender, about 10-12 minutes. When cauliflower is tender, remove the top of the steamer from the simmering water and place it over a bowl, so any excess water can drain out. Allow to cool, uncovered for about 10 minutes, then cover and place the steamer and the bowl in the refrigerator. Chill for at least 1/2 hour or until cool to the touch. While cauliflower is cooling, make the dressing. Pour olive oil in a small mixing bowl. Gradually stream in the lemon juice while vigorously whisking. Whisk in the garlic, mustard, sweetener, pepper, and salt.

In a medium mixing bowl, combine chilled cauliflower, peas, chives, almonds, and red onions. Pour dressing over and stir to mix. Transfer to an airtight container and refrigerate until serving. This salad is best if it is allowed to sit for a few hours in the refrigerator so the flavors mingle.

Nutrition Info

Calories: 212

Fat (g): 20

Carbs (g): 6

Fiber (g): 2 Protein (g):

Net Carbs (g): 4

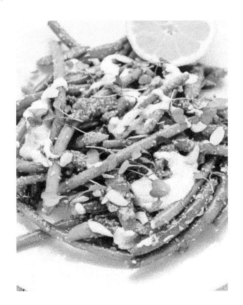

Black Bean Salad with Apricots

(Prep time: 15 min| Cooking Time: 15 min | serve: 2)

Ingredients

½ cup apricots, finely chopped

½ green bell pepper, finely chopped

¼ red onion, finely diced

½ cup black beans

½ cup finely chopped fresh rosemary

1/2 teaspoon ground cumin

Sea salt to taste

½ avocado, peeled, pitted, and chopped

2 tablespoons lime juice

2 teaspoons coconut oil

Lime juice

2 cups water

Instructions

Pour black beans and water into Instant Pot. Lock the lid into place. Select Pressure Cook or Manual, and adjust the pressure to High and the time to 10 minutes. After cooking, let the pressure release naturally for 2 minutes, then quickly release any remaining pressure.

Mix apricots, green bell pepper, and onions in a bowl; gently fold in black beans and rosemary. Season with ground cumin and sea salt. Fold in avocado and drizzle salad with lime juice and coconut oil. Let stand for 5-10 minutes before serving.

Nutrition Facts

Calories 426, Total Fat 17.7g, Saturated Fat 7.2g, Cholesterol 0mg, Sodium 133mg, Total Carbohydrate 53.6g, Dietary Fiber 18.5g, Total Sugars 7.2g, Protein 13.3g

Red Potato Salad
(Prep time: 5 min| Cooking Time: 20 min | serve: 2)

Ingredients

½ cup red potatoes or gold, cut into bite-sized pieces

1 egg

¼ cup mayonnaise

½ teaspoon Dijon mustard

¼ cup dill seed

1 small onion, thinly sliced

1 tablespoon cilantro, chopped

½ cup goat cheese, grated

1 teaspoon pepper

1 1/2 cups of water

Instructions

Pour 1 1/2 cups of water into the Instant Pot and insert the steam rack. Place cubed potatoes in a steamer basket and lower the steamer basket onto the steam rack. Add an egg on top of the potatoes.

Secure the lid, making sure the vent is closed.

Use the display panel and select the Manual or Pressure Cook function. Use the + /- keys and program the Instant Pot for 5 minutes.

When the time is up, quickly release the pressure.

Remove eggs and place in an ice bath. And the potatoes and allow to cool.

Keep the egg in an ice bath for 5 minutes, then peel and chop. Meanwhile, in a large bowl, whisk together mayonnaise and Dijon mustard. Mix in dill seed, onion, and cilantro. Fold in cooked potatoes, chopped eggs, goat cheese, and pepper. Season to taste.

Serve chilled garnish with extra cilantro.

Nutrition Facts

Calories 272, Total Fat 15.5g, Saturated Fat 3.3g, Cholesterol 93mg, Sodium 299mg, Total Carbohydrate 25.2g, Dietary Fiber 4.9g, Total Sugars 4.5g, Protein 8.1g

Awesome Pasta Salad

(Prep time: 30min| Cooking Time: 10 min | serve: 2)

Ingredients

½ cup fusilli pasta

½ cup cherry tomatoes halved

½ cup goat cheese, cubed

1 boiled egg

½ red bell pepper, cut into 1-inch pieces

½ cup corn, drained

½ cup mayonnaise

Salt and pepper to taste

¼ teaspoon oregano

½ teaspoon garlic powder

1 1/2 cups of water

Instructions

Put fusilli pasta in an Instant Pot. Stir in the water, oregano, garlic powder until smooth. Stir. Lock the lid onto the pot. Press Pressure Cook on Max Pressure for 5 minutes with the Keep Warm setting off.

When the Instant Pot has finished cooking, turn it off and let its pressure return naturally for 1 minute. Then use the Quick Release method to get rid of any residual pressure in the pot.

In a large bowl, combine pasta with cherry tomatoes, goat cheese, red bell pepper, egg, corn, and mayonnaise and toss to coat.

Nutrition Facts

Calories 227, Total Fat 8g, Saturated Fat 2.9g, Cholesterol 91mg, Sodium 194mg, Total Carbohydrate

29.1g, Dietary Fiber 2.8g, Total Sugars 5.2g, Protein 9.7g

Lemon-Mint Millet Salad

(Prep time: 15 min| Cooking Time: 15 min | serve: 2)

Ingredients

1 cup water

½ cup millet

1 lemon, zest, and juiced

½ cup roasted red peppers, drained and diced

¼ cup dried walnuts

1 tablespoon minced red onion

1 tablespoon chopped fresh mint

Instructions

Pour the millet into the Instant Pot. Add the water and kosher salt. Lock the lid into place. Select Pressure Cook or Manual, and adjust the pressure to High and the time to 10 minutes. After cooking, let the pressure release naturally for 2 minutes, then quickly release any remaining pressure. Unlock the lid. Remove the pot from the base. Fluff the millet with a fork and let it cool for a few minutes. Transfer it to a medium bowl.

Stir millet, lemon zest, and lemon juice together in a bowl. Add red peppers, walnuts, onions, and mint to millet; toss to combine.

Nutrition Facts

Calories 321, Total Fat 11.5g, Saturated Fat 0.9g, Cholesterol 0mg, Sodium 118mg, Total Carbohydrate 44.2g, Dietary Fiber 7g, Total Sugars 3.1g, Protein 10.2g

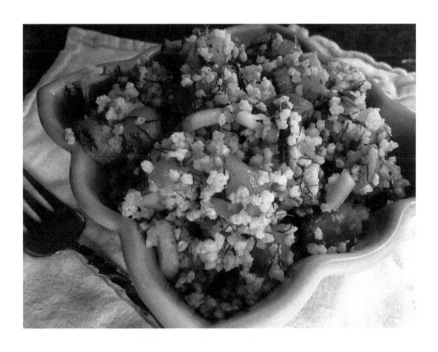

Beet and Carrot Barley Salad

(Prep time: 15 min| Cooking Time: 10 min | serve: 2)

Ingredients

1 cup water, or as needed

1 small beet, greens removed

½ cup barley

¼ teaspoon salt

2 ripened tomatoes, chopped

2 carrots, shredded

¼ bunch fresh mint, finely chopped

1 celery, chopped

1 lemon, zest, and juiced

Instructions

Pour the barley and beet into the Instant Pot. Add the water and kosher salt. Lock the lid into place. Select Pressure Cook or Manual, and adjust the pressure to

High and the time to 5 minutes. After cooking, let the pressure release naturally for 2 minutes, then quickly release any remaining pressure.

Unlock the lid. Stir Beet, barley mixture, tomatoes, carrots, mint, celery, lemon zest, and lemon juice together in a bowl; season with salt.

Nutrition Facts

Calories 260, Total Fat 1.5g, Saturated Fat 0.3g, Cholesterol 0mg, Sodium 109mg, Total Carbohydrate

53g, Dietary Fiber 13.2g, Total Sugars 11.6g, Protein 8.7g

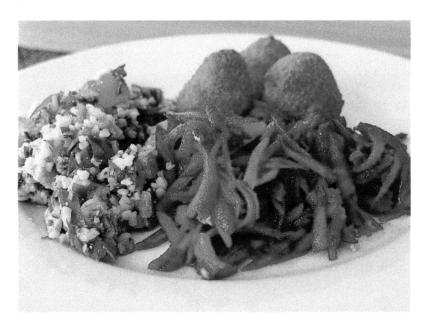

Quinoa, Asparagus, and Cucumber Salad

(Prep time: 15 min| Cooking Time: 10 min | serve: 2)

Ingredients

1 cup water

½ cup quinoa

½ cup thin asparagus spears, trimmed and cut into 1-inch

1 cucumber, peeled, seeded, and chopped

1 leek, chopped

½ tablespoon Dijon mustard

¼ tablespoon honey

½ tablespoon olive oil

1/4 cup chopped fresh basil

2 heads butter lettuce

Salt and pepper to taste

Instructions

Pour the quinoa and asparagus into the Instant Pot. Add the water and kosher salt. Lock the lid into place. Select Pressure Cook or Manual, and adjust the pressure to High and the time to 5 minutes. After cooking, let the pressure release naturally for 2 minutes, then quickly release any remaining pressure. Unlock the lid.

Whisk together the honey, Dijon mustard, olive oil, and chopped basil. Cover salad and dressing separately. Refrigerate until chilled.

Pour dressing into quinoa, asparagus mixture with cucumber, leek, and season with salt and pepper. Line a large bowl with lettuce and mound salad in a bowl. Garnish with basil sprigs.

Nutrition Facts

Calories 320, Total Fat 7.3g, Saturated Fat 0.9g, Cholesterol 0mg, Sodium 86mg, Total Carbohydrate

53.1g, Dietary Fiber 7.7g, Total Sugars 10.3g, Protein 10.5g

Wild Rice Salad with Tofu

(Prep time: 20 min| Cooking Time: 10 min | serve: 2)

Ingredients

¼ cup wild rice

½ cup light mayonnaise

¼ teaspoon red vinegar

¼ teaspoon maple syrup

Salt and pepper to taste

½ cup cubed tofu

¼ cup diced leek

1/8 cup seedless raisins

¼ cup walnut

1small onion, thinly sliced

Instructions

Pour the wild rice into Instant Pot. Add the water. Lock the lid into place. Select Pressure Cook or Manual, and adjust the pressure to High and the time to 5 minutes. After cooking, let the pressure release naturally for 2 minutes, then quickly release any remaining pressure. In a medium bowl, whisk together the mayonnaise, vinegar, maple syrup, salt, and pepper.

Stir in rice, tofu, onion, and raisins, leeks until evenly coated with dressing. Cover and refrigerate for 1- 2 hours. Before serving, sprinkle walnut over the top of the salad.

Nutrition Facts

Calories 552, Total Fat 34.6g, Saturated Fat 4.2g, Cholesterol 15mg, Sodium 432mg, Total

Carbohydrate 42.6g, Dietary Fiber 4.3g, Total Sugars 10.7g, Protein 17.6g

Buckwheat Salad with Mint, Walnuts, and Cranberries

(Prep time: 25 min| Cooking Time: 10 min | serve: 2)

Ingredients

½ cup buckwheat

½ tablespoon coconut oil

¼ cup coarsely chopped mint leaves

¼ cup dry-roasted walnuts, unsalted

1/8 cup dried cranberries

¼ cup chopped spinach

¼ cup sliced carrots

¼ cup sliced leek

1small onion, thinly sliced

1 tomato, halved

½ lemon zest, juiced

Salt and ground black pepper to taste

1 cup water

Instructions

Pour the buckwheat into Instant Pot. Add the water. Lock the lid into place. Select Pressure Cook or Manual, and adjust the pressure to High and the time to 5 minutes. After cooking, let the pressure release naturally for 2 minutes, then quickly release any remaining pressure.

Stir coconut oil, mint, walnuts, dried cranberries, spinach, carrots, leeks, onions, tomatoes, lemon juice, and lemon zest. Season to taste with salt and ground black pepper.

Serve.

Nutrition Facts

Calories 342, Total Fat 14.3g, Saturated Fat 3.8g, Cholesterol 0mg, Sodium 20mg, Total Carbohydrate

42.6g, Dietary Fiber 8.1g, Total Sugars 5g, Protein 10.9g

Dinner

Peanut Chutney Mushrooms with Tamarind

(Prep time: 15 min |Cooking Time: 15 min | serve: 2)

Ingredients

1 1/2 tablespoons olive oil, divided

½ cup raw peanuts

1 dried red Chile

½ tablespoon cumin seeds

½ tablespoon coriander seeds

5 curry leaves torn into pieces

½ teaspoon kosher salt, divided

1 tablespoon tamarind concentrate

Water

2 onions, diced

½ teaspoon ginger powder

½ teaspoon garlic powder

1 cup mushrooms cut into 1-inch pieces

Instructions

Using the Sauté function on High, heat 1 tablespoon oil in the Instant Pot for about 1 minute, until shimmering. Add the peanuts and cook for 1 minute, frequently stirring, until fragrant. Add the chilies, cumin seeds, coriander seeds, and curry leaves; cook for 1 minute until fragrant. Transfer the nuts and spices to a blender and let cool slightly. Remove 1/4 cup of the peanut mixture and set aside. Add 1 teaspoon salt and the tamarind concentrate to the blender; blend on high speed until smooth, adding 1 tablespoon water if needed to help the mixture blend. Using the Sauté function on High, heat 2 tablespoons of oil in the Instant Pot for about 1 minute, until shimmering. Add the onions and cook for about 4 minutes, occasionally stirring, until softened. Add the ginger and garlic; cook for about 1 minute, until fragrant.

Stir in the mushrooms, 1/2 cup water, peanut chutney, and remaining 1 teaspoon salt. Secure the lid and cook on High Pressure for 8 minutes.

Once the cooking is complete, let the pressure release naturally for 10 minutes, then quick-release the remaining pressure. Transfer the curry to a platter. Pour the reserved peanuts and spices over the mushrooms and serve.

Nutrition Facts

Calories 353, Total Fat 26.3g, Saturated Fat 3.6g, Cholesterol 0mg, Sodium 65mg, Total Carbohydrate

24.1g, Dietary Fiber 8g, Total Sugars 9.2g, Protein 12.9g

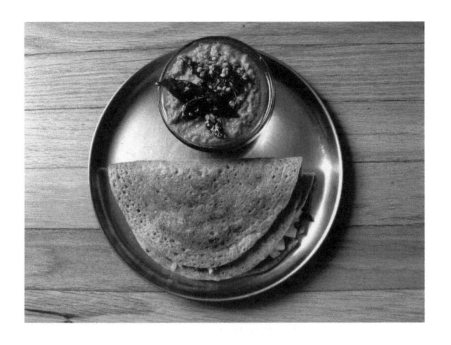

Tofu with 20 Cloves of Garlic

(Prep time: 5 min |Cooking Time: 25 min | serve: 2)

Ingredients

2 cups tofu cut into pieces

1/4 teaspoon sea salt

½ tablespoon coconut oil

20 cloves garlic or more

½ teaspoon basil, chopped

½ teaspoon rosemary, chopped

½ teaspoon thyme, chopped

½ cup vegetable stock

1 tablespoon coconut cream

1 tablespoon arrowroot

Instructions

Season the pieces of tofu with sea salt. Select the Sauté setting on your Instant Pot, allowing it to come up to temperature. Add ¼ tablespoon of coconut oil to the Instant Pot, and swirl around. Add half of the tofu pieces, and sear on the other side for 4 minutes. Set this tofu aside, and repeat with the remaining tofu. Add the garlic cloves to the Instant Pot, and sauté for 1-2 minutes, stirring frequently. Turn off the Sauté setting. Add the tofu back into the Instant Pot and sprinkle it liberally with the chopped herbs. Add the vegetable stock to the Instant Pot, then seal the lid. Select High, and set a time for 10 minutes. Once the timer has gone off, allow the Instant Pot to depressurize for about 10 minutes gradually. Remove the tofu and set it aside to keep warm. Turn the Sauté function back on High. Add the coconut cream to the Instant Pot with the stock and garlic and stir gently. Dilute the arrowroot in some water and stir in gradually to thicken the sauce. After it has thickened to a rich consistency, pour the creamy garlic clove sauce over the tofu and serve.

Nutrition Facts

Calories 272, Total Fat 15.9g, Saturated Fat 6.7g, Cholesterol 0mg, Sodium 284mg, Total Carbohydrate 15.4g, Dietary Fiber 3.3g, Total Sugars 2.2g, Protein 23g

Mushrooms and Olive Curry

(Prep time: 15 min |Cooking Time: 15 min | serve: 2)

Ingredients

1 teaspoon red chili powder

½ teaspoon ground cumin

½ teaspoon turmeric powder

¼ teaspoon ground ginger

1/8 teaspoon ground cinnamon

2 cups mushrooms

Salt and pepper to taste

2 tablespoons vegetable oil

1 onion sliced

1 teaspoon garlic powder

1 tablespoon tomato paste

1 cup vegetable broth

¼ lemon juiced

¼ cup high-quality pitted olives

Instructions

Combine the red chili powder, cumin, turmeric, ginger powder, and cinnamon in a small bowl. Season the mushrooms generously with salt and pepper on it. Place in a bowl or plastic bag to marinate for at least 1 hour.

Once the mushrooms are done marinating, turn on the Sauté function of Instant Pot. Once hot, add the vegetable oil. Add mushrooms, and cook for about 3 minutes without moving. Set aside. Add the onion and cook for 2 minutes, scraping the bottom of the Instant Pot. Add the garlic powder and tomato paste and cook, stirring for 1 more minute. Turn off the Sauté function. Add the broth and scrape any remaining bits off the bottom of the Instant Pot. Add the mushrooms, and squeeze them in so that they fit in one layer. Secure the lid. Cook at High Pressure for 5 minutes and use a natural release. Remove the mushrooms and some of the onions. Turn on the Sauté function and simmer the sauce for 10 to 15 minutes, until reduced by more than half and starting to thicken. Turn off the Sauté function. Add the lemon juice, stir, and taste for seasoning. To serve, pour the sauce over the mushrooms and sprinkle the olives on top.

Nutrition Facts

Calories 199, Total Fat 16.8g, Saturated Fat 3.2g, Cholesterol 0mg, Sodium 555mg, Total Carbohydrate 9.3g, Dietary Fiber 2.8g, Total Sugars 3.5g, Protein 5.8g

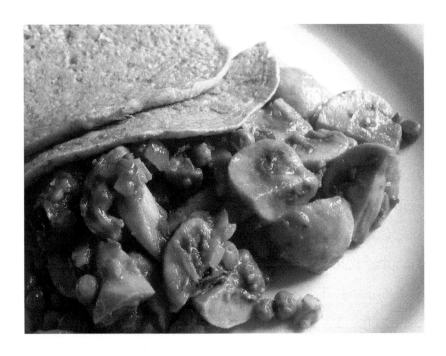

Baked Kohlrabi Yucca Root and Mustard Greens

Ingredients

1/2 pound kohlrabi, cut into chunks

½ pound yucca root, cut into chunks

½ pound mustard greens

2 tablespoons extra virgin olive oil

12 cloves garlic, thinly sliced

1 tbsp. and 1 tsp. dried rosemary

4 teaspoons dried thyme

2 teaspoons sea salt

1 bunch fresh green beans, trimmed and cut

Directions:

Preheat your oven to 425 degrees F. In a baking pan, combine the first 7 ingredients and 1/2 of the sea salt. Cover with foil. Bake 20 minutes in the oven. Combine the green beans, olive oil, and salt. Cover, and cook for about 15 minutes, or until the root vegetables become tender. Take out the foil, and cook for 8 minutes until potatoes become lightly browned.

Baked Brussel Sprouts & Red Onion Glazed with Balsamic Vinegar

Ingredients

1 (16 ounces) package fresh Brussels sprouts

2 small red onions, thinly sliced

¼ cup and 1 tbsp. extra-virgin olive oil, divided

1/4 teaspoon sea salt

1/4 teaspoon rainbow peppercorns

1 shallot, chopped

1/4 cup balsamic vinegar

1 tablespoon chopped fresh rosemary

Directions:

Preheat your oven to 425 degrees F (220 degrees C). Grease a baking pan.

Combine Brussels sprouts and onion in a bowl. Add 4 tablespoons of olive oil, salt, and peppercorns. Toss to coat and spread the sprout mixture on the pan. Bake in the oven until sprouts and red onion becomes tender, for about 25 to 30 minutes. Heat the remaining tablespoon of olive oil in a small skillet over medium-high heat Sauté the shallots until tender, for about 5 minutes. Add balsamic vinegar and cook until the glaze is reduced for about 5 minutes. Add rosemary into the balsamic glaze and pour over the sprouts.

Baked Purple Cabbage with Rainbow Peppercorns

Ingredients

1 (16 ounces) package fresh purple cabbage

2 small red onions, thinly sliced

1/2 cup and 1 tbsp. extra-virgin olive oil, divided

1/4 teaspoon sea salt

1/4 teaspoon rainbow peppercorns

1 shallot, chopped

1/4 cup balsamic vinegar

1 tsp. herbs de Provence

Directions:

Preheat your oven to 425 degrees F (220 degrees C). Grease a baking pan. Combine cabbage and onion in a bowl. Add 4 tablespoons of olive oil, salt, and peppercorns. Toss to coat and spread the sprouts mixture on the pan. Bake in the oven until sprouts and onion become tender, for about 25 to 30 minutes. Heat the remaining tablespoon of olive oil in a small skillet over medium-high heat Sauté the shallots until tender, for about 5 minutes. Add balsamic vinegar and cook until the glaze is reduced for about 5 minutes. Add herbs de Provence into the balsamic glaze and pour over the sprouts.

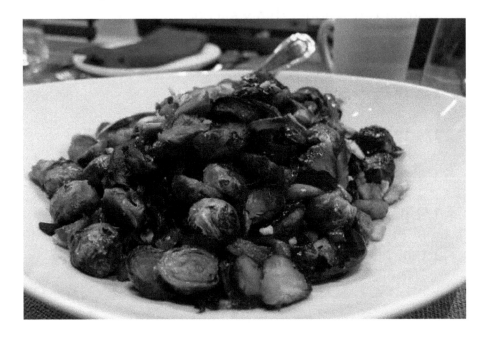

Roasted Microgreens and Potatoes

Ingredients

1 ½ pounds potatoes, peeled and cut into 1-inch chunks

½ onion, thinly sliced

¼ cup water

½ vegetable stock cube, crumbled

1 tbsp. olive oil

½ tsp minced ginger

2 sprigs of lemon grass

½ tsp green onions, minced

½ tsp hot chili powder

Black pepper

½ pound Microgreens, roughly chopped

Directions:

Put all of the ingredients in a slow cooker except the last one. Top with handfuls of Microgreens and stuff the slow cooker with it. If you can't fit it all in at once, let

the first batch cook first and add some more
Microgreens. Cook for 3or 4 hours on medium until
potatoes become soft. Scrape the sides and serve.

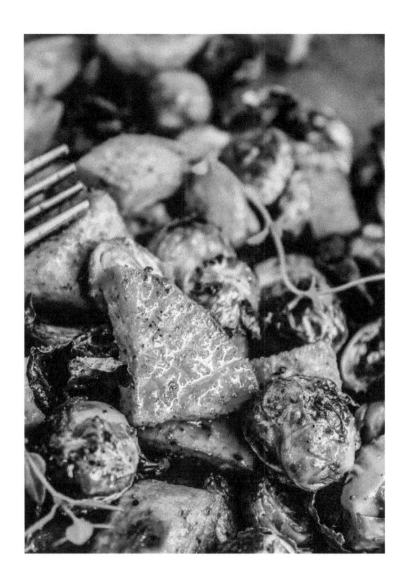

Roasted Spinach & Broccoli with Jalapeno

Ingredients

1 ½ pound broccoli florets

½ onion, thinly sliced

¼ cup water

½ vegetable stock cube, crumbled

1 tbsp. extra virgin olive oil

½ tsp cumin

8 jalapeno peppers, finely chopped

1 ancho chili

½ tsp hot chili powder

Black pepper

½ pound fresh spinach, roughly chopped

Directions:

Put all of the ingredients in a slow cooker except the last one. Top with handfuls of spinach and stuff the slow cooker with it. If you can't fit it all in at once, let the first batch cook first and add some more spinach. Cook for 3or 4 hours on medium until broccoli becomes soft. Scrape the sides and serve.

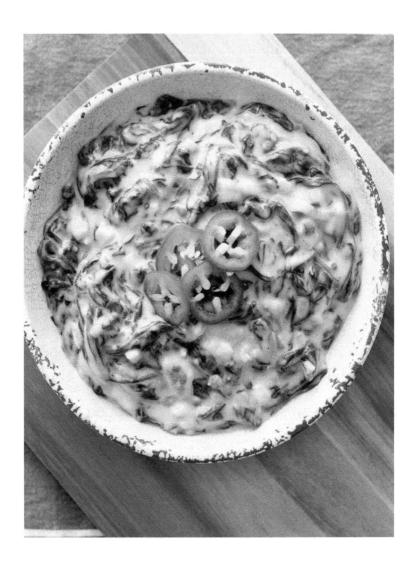

Spicy Baked Swiss Chard and Cauliflower

Ingredients

1 ½ pound cauliflower florets, blanched (dipped in boiling water then dipped in ice water)

½ cup bean sprouts, rinsed

½ cup water

½ vegetable stock cube, crumbled

1 tbsp. sesame oil

½ tsp Thai chili paste

½ tsp Sriracha hot sauce

½ tsp hot chili powder

2 Thai bird chilies, minced Black pepper

½ pound fresh Swiss chard, roughly chopped

Directions:

Put all of the ingredients in a slow cooker except the last one. Top with handfuls of Swiss chard and stuff the slow cooker with it. If you can't fit it all in at once, let the first batch cook first and add some more Swiss chard. Cook for 3 or 4 hours on medium until potatoes become soft. Scrape the sides and serve.

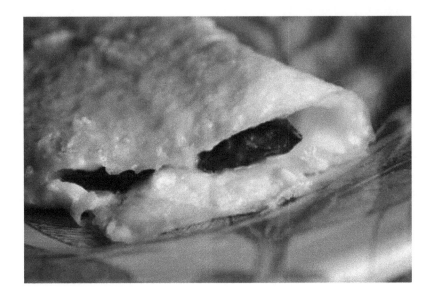

Thai Carrots and Collard Greens

Ingredients

1 ½ pounds carrots, peeled and cut into 1-inch chunks

½ onion, thinly sliced

¼ cup water

½ vegetable stock cube, crumbled

1 tbsp. extra virgin olive oil

1 tbsp. sesame oil

½ tsp Thai chili paste

½ tsp Sriracha hot sauce

½ tsp hot chili powder

2 Thai bird chilies, minced Black pepper

½ pound collard greens, roughly chopped

Directions:

Put all of the ingredients in a slow cooker except the last one. Top with handfuls of collard greens and stuff the slow cooker with it. If you can't fit it all in at once, let the first batch cook first and add some more collard greens. Cook for 3or 4 hours on medium until carrots become soft. Scrape the sides and serve.

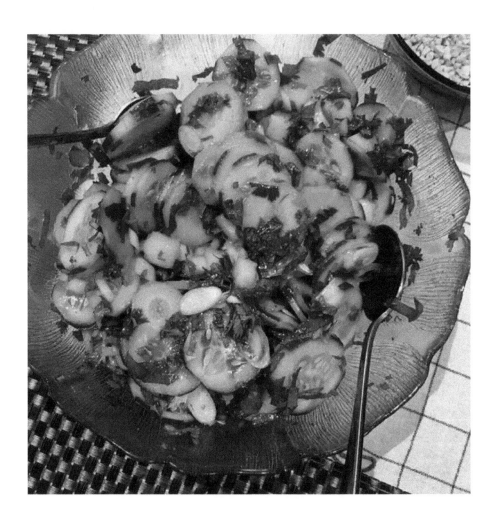

Baked White Yam and Spinach

Ingredients

½ pounds potatoes, peeled and cut into 1-inch chunks

½ pounds white yam, peeled and cut into 1-inch chunks

½ pounds carrots, peeled and cut into 1- inch chunks

½ red onion, thinly sliced

¼ cup water

½ vegetable stock cube, crumbled

1 tbsp. extra virgin olive oil

½ tsp cumin

½ tsp ground coriander

½ tsp garam masala

½ tsp cayenne pepper Black pepper

½ pound fresh spinach, roughly chopped

Directions:

Put all of the ingredients in a slow cooker except the last one. Top with handfuls of spinach and stuff the slow cooker with it. If you can't fit it all in at once, let the first batch cook first and add some more spinach. Cook for 3or 4 hours on medium until potatoes become soft. Scrape the sides and serve.

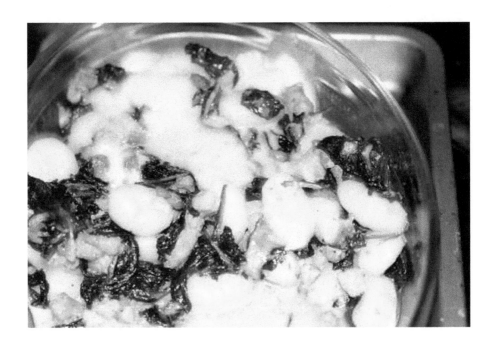

Sweets

Carrot Oatmeal Muffins

Prep time: 30 min Cooking Time: 20 min serve: 2

Ingredients

½ cup almond flour

¼ cup coconut flour

½ teaspoons baking soda

½ teaspoon baking powder

¼ teaspoon salt

¼ teaspoon cinnamon

1 tablespoon honey

1 cup coconut oil

1 egg, beaten

½ teaspoon vanilla extract

¼ cup uncooked rolled oats

¼ cup flaked coconut

½ tablespoon raisins

½ cup shredded carrots

¼ cup crushed pineapple

Instructions

In a large bowl, mix the almond flour, coconut flour, baking soda, baking powder, salt, and cinnamon. Make a well in the centre of the mixture, and add honey, coconut oil, egg, and vanilla. Mix just until evenly moist. Fold in the oats, coconut flour, raisins, carrots, and pineapple.

Fill each muffin cup is about 2/3 full.

Place the pan onto the trivet and cover loosely with aluminium foil. Close the lid, set the Pressure Release to Sealing, and select Manual/Pressure Cook. Set the Instant Pot to 20 minutes on High Pressure and let cook.

Once cooked, let the pressure release naturally from the Instant Pot for about 10 minutes, then carefully switch the Pressure Release to Venting.

Open the Instant Pot and remove the pan. Let cool, serve and enjoy!

Nutrition Facts

Calories 379, Total Fat 22.8g, Saturated Fat 6.9g, Cholesterol 82mg , Sodium 664mg, Total Carbohydrate 32.4g, Dietary Fiber 6.8g, Total Sugars 15.5g, Protein 11.2g

Banana Blueberry Muffins

Prep time: 30 min Cooking Time: 20 min serve: 2

Ingredients

½ cup flax meal

½ tablespoon honey

1/8 teaspoon ground cinnamon

¼ teaspoons baking powder

¼ teaspoon baking soda

1 mashed banana

1 egg white

1/8 teaspoon vanilla extract

1 tablespoon fresh blueberries

1 cup water

Instructions

Mix the flax meal, honey, cinnamon, baking powder, and baking soda. In a separate bowl, mix the banana, egg white, and vanilla extract.

Mix the banana mixture into the flour mixture until smooth. Fold in the blueberries. Spoon the batter into the pan prepared for the muffins.

Pour 1 cup water into the Instant Pot. Place the trivet inside. Place the muffin cups on the rack or pan.

Secure the lid and set the Pressure Release valve to Sealing. Press the Pressure Cook or Manual button and set the cook time to 20 minutes.

When the Instant Pot beeps, allow the pressure to release naturally for 10 minutes, then carefully switch the Pressure Release valve to Venting. When fully released, open the lid. Carefully remove the muffins. Allow them to cool for about 15 minutes.

Nutrition Facts

Calories 233, Total Fat 10.2g, Saturated Fat 0.1g, Cholesterol 0mg , Sodium 177mg, Total Carbohydrate 27g, Dietary Fiber 9.7g , Total Sugars 12.1g, Protein 8.5g

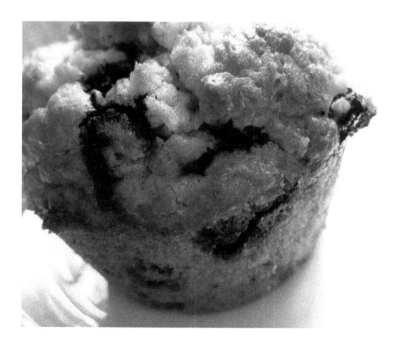

Lemon Zucchini Muffins

Prep time: 15 min Cooking Time: 25 min serve: 2

Ingredients

½ cup coconut flour

2 tablespoons honey

¼ teaspoon baking powder

¼ teaspoon baking soda

1/8 teaspoon salt

½ zucchini, shredded

¼ cup lemon yogurt

2 tablespoons butter, melted

1 egg, beaten

1 tablespoon lemon juice

1 tablespoon lemon zest

1 cup water

Instructions

Mix flour, honey, baking powder, baking soda, and salt in a large bowl; make a well in the centre of the flour mixture. Mix zucchini, yogurt, butter, egg, 1 tablespoon lemon juice, and 1 tablespoon lemon zest in a separate bowl; pour yogurt mixture into well.

Pour 1 cup water into the Instant Pot. Place the trivet inside. Place the muffin cups on the rack or pan.

Secure the lid and set the Pressure Release valve to Sealing. Press the Pressure Cook or Manual button and set the cook time to 20 minutes.

When the Instant Pot beeps, allow the pressure to release naturally for 10 minutes, then carefully switch the Pressure Release valve to Venting. When fully released, open the lid. Carefully remove the muffins. Allow them to cool for about 15 minutes.

Nutrition Facts

Calories 244, Total Fat 14.7g, Saturated Fat 8.8g, Cholesterol 114mg, Sodium 455mg, Total Carbohydrate 23.8g, Dietary Fiber 1.9g, Total Sugars 20.8g, Protein 5.8g

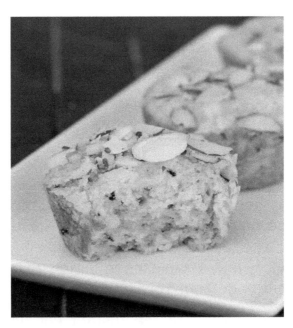

Banana Chocolate Chip Muffins

Prep time: 15 min Cooking Time: 20 min serve: 2

Ingredients

½ cup almond flour

1 tablespoon honey

½ teaspoon cocoa powder

1/8 tablespoon baking powder

1 mashed banana

½ teaspoon olive oil

1 egg, beaten

1tablespoon semi-sweet chocolate chips

1 cup water

Instructions

In a large bowl combine the flour, honey, cocoa powder and baking powder.

In another bowl, blend the banana, oil and egg. Add to dry ingredients, mixing just until blended. Fold in the chocolate chips.

Pour 1 cup water into the Instant Pot. Place the trivet inside. Place the muffin cups on the rack or pan.

Secure the lid and set the Pressure Release valve to Sealing. Press the Pressure Cook or Manual button and set the cook time to 20 minutes.

When the Instant Pot beeps, allow the pressure to release naturally for 10 minutes, then carefully switch the Pressure Release valve to Venting. When fully released, open the lid. Carefully remove the muffins. Allow them to cool for about 15 minutes.

Nutrition Facts

Calories 189, Total Fat 10.5g, Saturated Fat 1.5g, Cholesterol 41mg, Sodium 39mg, Total Carbohydrate 18.7g, Dietary Fiber 2.6g, Total Sugars 11.2g, Protein 5g

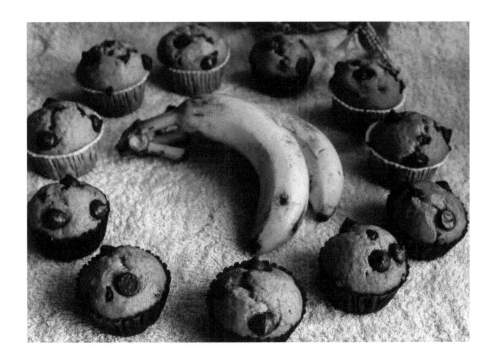

Brownie Muffins
Servings 6

Ingredients

1 cup golden flaxseed meal

¼ cup cocoa powder

1 tablespoon cinnamon

½ tablespoon baking powder

½ teaspoon salt 1 large egg

2 tablespoons coconut oil

¼ cup sugar-free caramel syrup

½ cup pumpkin puree

1 teaspoon vanilla extract

1 teaspoon apple cider vinegar

¼ cup slivered almonds

Instructions

Preheat your oven to 350°F and combine all your dry ingredients in a deep mixing bowl and mix to combine.

In a separate bowl, combine all your wet ingredients.

Pour your wet ingredients into your dry ingredients and mix very well to combine.

Line a muffin tin with paper liners and spoon about ¼ cup of batter into each muffin liner. This recipe should Servings 6 muffins. Then sprinkle slivered almonds over the top of each muffin and press gently so that they adhere.

Bake in the oven for about 15 minutes. You should see the muffins rise and set on top. Enjoy warm or cool!

Nutrition Info

193 Calories 14.09g Fats 4.37g Net Carbs 6.98g Protein.

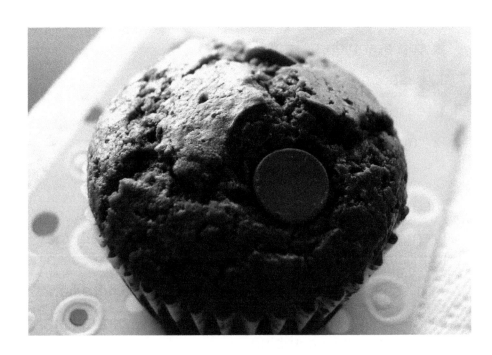

Milkshake ice pops

Prep:10 mins plus 4 hrs freezing, no cook easy Makes 4

Ingredients

405ml can light condensed milk

1 tsp vanilla bean paste

1 ripe chopped banana

10 strawberries or 3 tbsp chocolate hazelnut spread

Directions:

Pour the light condensed milk into a food processor and add the vanilla bean paste and chopped banana. Whizz until smooth. Add either the strawberries or chocolate hazelnut spread and whizz again.

Divide the mixture between 4 paper cups, cover with foil, then push a lolly stick through the foil lid of each cup until you hit the base. Freeze for 4 hrs or until solid. Will keep in the freezer for 2 months.

Whisky & pink peppercorn marmalade kit Easy

Ingredients

500g mix of oranges, clementines and lemons

1kg demerara sugar

small pot of pink peppercorns

small bottle of whisky

Optional extras

jam pan muslin large wooden spoon

small jars and labels (makes about 1kg jam)

Directions:

To use the kit:

Write the following instructions on the gift tag:Halve the fruits and squeeze the juices into a large saucepan. Remove all the peel and set aside. Put the flesh in the pan with 1 litre water and boil for 15 mins. Push through a sieve lined with muslin and return the liquid to the pan.

Shred the peel and tip into a heatproof bowl. Add enough water to just cover and microwave for 3-4 mins until soft. Add the peel to the pan, then add the sugar. Boil for 35-45 mins until the marmalade has reached setting point (keep an eye on it so it doesn't bubble over).

Remove from the heat and add 1 tsp pink peppercorns. Allow the mixture to cool a little, then stir in 50ml whisky. Ladle into sterilised jars and seal. Will keep for up to one year.

Simnel muffins

Prep:45 mins - 55 mins easy Makes 12

Ingredients

250g mixed dried fruit

grated zest and juice 1 medium orange

175g softened butter

175g golden caster sugar

3 eggs , beaten

300g self-raising flour

1 tsp mixed spice

½ tsp freshly grated nutmeg

5 tbsp milk

175g marzipan

200g icing sugar

2 tbsp orange juice for mixing

mini eggs

Directions:

Tip the fruit into a bowl, add the zest and juice and microwave on medium for 2 minutes (or leave to soak for 1 hour). Line 12 deep muffin tins with paper muffin cases.

Preheat the oven to fan 180C/ 160C/gas

Beat the butter, sugar, eggs, flour, spices and milk until light and fluffy (about 3-5 minutes) – use a wooden spoon or hand held mixer. Stir the fruit in well. Half fill the muffin cases with the mixture. Divide the marzipan into 12 equal pieces, roll into balls, then flatten with your thumb to the size of the muffin cases. Put one into each muffin case and spoon the rest of the mixture over it. Bake for 25-30 minutes, until risen, golden and firm to the touch. Leave to cool.

Beat together the icing sugar and orange juice to make icing thick enough to coat the back of a wooden spoon. Drizzle over the muffins and top with a cluster of eggs. Leave to set. Best eaten within a day of making.

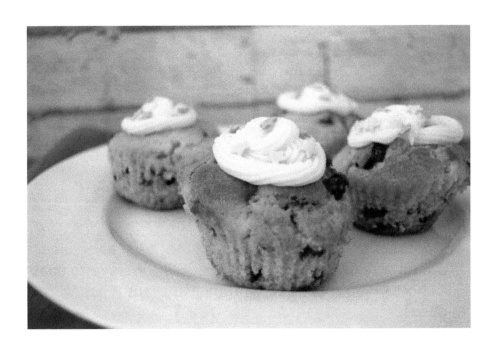

Prunes Cake

Prep time:20 min Cooking Time: 50min serve: 2

Ingredients

¼ cup vegetable oil

¼ cup honey

1 egg

2 cups coconut flour

½ teaspoon salt

1 teaspoon baking powder

1 cup coconut milk

1 teaspoon vanilla extract

¼ teaspoon almond extract

2 cups chopped prunes, divided

¼ cup water

1 tablespoon lemon juice

Instructions

Spray two 8-inch round cake pans with vegetable oil spray.

In a medium bowl, sift together coconut flour, salt and baking powder. Set aside.

In a large mixing bowl, making cream add vegetable oil with the honey until fluffy. Add egg and beat well. Add flour mixture coconut milk. Fold in vanilla and almond extracts and 1 cup chopped prunes.

Pour water into Instant Pot. Place wire trivet into the bottom of the pot and set the pan on top. Place lid on pot and lock into place to seal. Pressure Cook or Manual on High Pressure for 30 minutes. Let sit 10 minutes. Use Quick Pressure Release. Keep cake aside.

To make the filling: In an Instant pot, combine reaming chopped prunes, honey, and water and lemon juice. Close the lid of Instant pot, Pressure Cook or Manual on High Pressure for 20 minutes. Let sit 10 minutes. Use Quick Pressure Release. Spread thinly between cooled cake layers and on top.

Nutrition Facts

Calories 316, Total Fat 23.9g, Saturated Fat 12.7g, Cholesterol 33mg, Sodium 256mg, Total Carbohydrate 77.2g, Dietary Fiber 4.9g, Total Sugars 28.9g, Protein 8.2g

Butternut squash. -Almond Cookies

Prep time: 40 min Cooking Time: 25 min serve: 2

Ingredients

1 cup butter, soften

¼ cup honey

1 egg, beaten

¼ teaspoon vanilla extract

1 cup butternut squash. puree

2 cups coconut flour

1 teaspoon baking powder

1 teaspoon baking soda

¼ teaspoon salt

1 teaspoon ground nutmeg

¼ cup walnuts

Instructions

Line the Instant Pot with parchment paper and spray with nonstick coconut oil spray. Set aside.

Cream together the butter and honey.

Beat together the egg, vanilla and butternut squash puree.

Sift together the coconut flour, baking powder, baking soda, salt and nutmeg; combine with butternut squash mixture and stir in almond.

Add the cookie dough to the prepared Instant pot. Using a rubber spatula, spread and press the dough into the bottom of the pot, making sure to cover the bottom completely and filling in any gaps.

Cover and lock the lid, but leave the steam release handle in the Venting position. Select High pressure and set the cook time for 15 min. When the cook time is complete, press Cancel to turn off the pot.

Open the lid and carefully transfer the inner pot with the cookie to a cooling rack. Allow the cookie to cool in the pot for a minimum of 30 minutes or until it reaches room temperature.

Nutrition Facts

Calories 193, Total Fat 17.4g, Saturated Fat 10g, Cholesterol 54mg , Sodium 270mg, Total Carbohydrate 8.1g, Dietary Fiber 0.8g , Total Sugars 6.6g, Protein 1.5g

Lightning Source UK Ltd.
Milton Keynes UK
UKHW050320110521
383304UK00004B/61